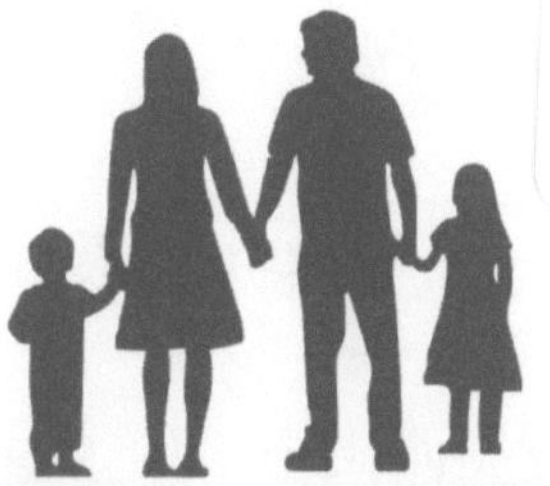

EVER FOUND YOURSELF CHASING RUNAWAY TOYS WHILE SIMULTANEOUSLY NEGOTIATING A PEACE TREATY BETWEEN ARGUING SIBLINGS, ALL BEFORE YOUR MORNING COFFEE HAS HAD A CHANCE TO KICK IN? IF YOU'RE NODDING WITH THE WEARIED RECOGNITION OF A PARENT WHO'S BEEN THERE, WELCOME TO A SPACE THAT UNDERSTANDS THE DAILY JUGGLING ACT OF PARENTHOOD. IN THE CHAOTIC ORCHESTRA OF SPILLED CEREAL, MISPLACED HOMEWORK, AND UNTIED SHOELACES, WE'VE ALL YEARNED FOR A PAUSE BUTTON—A CHANCE TO BREATHE AND SAVOR THE SWEET MADNESS THAT IS RAISING KIDS. "CALM AND CONNECTED: NAVIGATING PARENTHOOD MINDFULLY" INVITES YOU INTO A JOURNEY THAT DOESN'T PROMISE TO ELIMINATE THE CHAOS BUT PROMISES SOMETHING EVEN BETTER: THE ABILITY TO FIND CALM WITHIN IT. PICTURE A GUIDEBOOK THAT TURNS SPILLED MILK INTO AN OPPORTUNITY FOR LAUGHTER AND SIBLING SQUABBLES INTO LESSONS IN EMPATHY. READY TO EMBRACE A MINDFUL APPROACH THAT'S AS REAL AND MESSY AS YOUR MORNING ROUTINE?

Mindfulness is awareness of one's internal states and surroundings.
- American Psychological Association

CONTENTS

Chapter 1: Welcome to Mindful Parenting

Chapter 2: Mindfulness Demystified

Chapter 3: The Science Behind Mindful Parenting

Chapter 4: Creating Mindful Moments

Chapter 5: Mindful Breathing Techniques

Chapter 6: Responding vs. Reacting

Chapter 7: Managing Parental Stress Mindfully

Chapter 8: The Art of Presence

Chapter 9: Communicating Mindfully

Chapter 10: Creating a Mindful Home

Chapter 11: Mindful Rituals and Traditions

Chapter 12: Overcoming Challenges and Staying Mindful

Chapter 13: Growing Together Mindfully

CHAPTER 1: WELCOME TO MINDFUL PARENTING

OVERVIEW:

Welcome to a transformative journey where the ordinary moments of parenthood become extraordinary through the lens of mindfulness. In this chapter, we'll explore the essence of mindful parenting and set the foundation for a parenting style that embraces calm amidst chaos. Brace yourself for a refreshing perspective that turns everyday challenges into opportunities for connection and joy.

THE MINDFUL PARENTING PARADIGM:

Mindful parenting isn't about achieving a mythical state of perpetual tranquility but rather about being present in each moment, no matter how mundane or chaotic. Picture this: your child excitedly shares a school story, and instead of mentally multitasking, you immerse yourself in the joy of their narrative. This paradigm shift is the heart of mindful parenting.

CHAPTER 1: WELCOME TO MINDFUL PARENTING

THE POWER OF PRESENCE:

One of the foundational principles of mindful parenting is the power of presence. It's about showing up mentally and emotionally, fully engaged in the now. Whether it's bath time, bedtime stories, or a spontaneous game of catch, the act of being fully present fosters a deeper connection with your child.

MINDFULNESS IN ACTION:

To kickstart your mindful parenting journey, try incorporating a brief mindfulness exercise into your daily routine. Begin with a simple breathing exercise, taking a few moments to focus on your breath. Notice the rise and fall of your chest, and let go of any tension. This exercise is your anchor to the present moment.

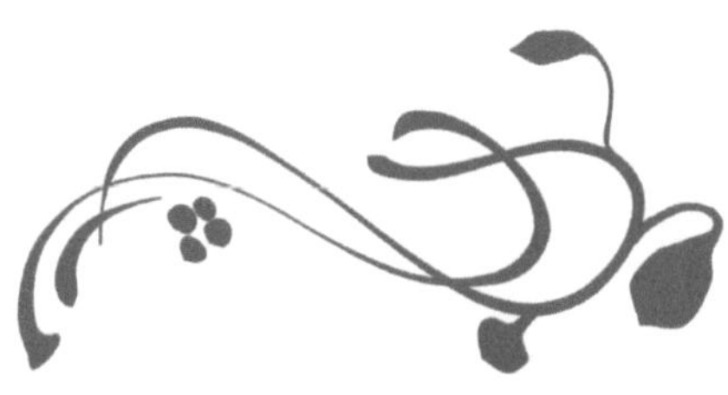

CHAPTER 1: WELCOME TO MINDFUL PARENTING

YOUR MINDFUL PARENTING JOURNAL:

As you embark on this journey, consider keeping a mindful parenting journal. Document your observations, thoughts, and the small victories that arise from being present. This journal will serve as a valuable reflection tool and a reminder of your growth as a mindful parent.

NEXT STEPS:

Are you ready to infuse mindfulness into your parenting journey? In the next chapter, we'll demystify the concept of mindfulness and explore its profound impact on both you and your child. Get ready to discover how the simple act of being present can revolutionize your parenting experience.

CHAPTER 2: MINDFULNESS DEMYSTIFIED

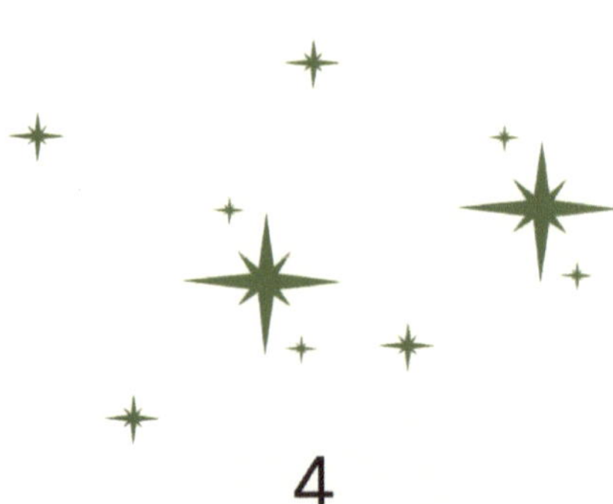

DEMYSTIFYING MINDFULNESS:

Now that you've taken your first steps into the world of mindful parenting, let's dive deeper into the concept of mindfulness itself. At its core, mindfulness is about cultivating awareness and attention to the present moment without judgment. It's not about eliminating thoughts or achieving a perfect state but rather about acknowledging and observing them.

THE MINDFUL PARENT'S TOOLKIT:

As a mindful parent, consider your awareness as a powerful toolkit. Picture it filled with tools like patience, compassion, and non-reactivity. These tools are readily available to you, enhancing your ability to respond thoughtfully to your child's needs, rather than reacting impulsively.

CHAPTER 2: MINDFULNESS DEMYSTIFIED

INCORPORATING MINDFULNESS INTO DAILY LIFE:

Mindfulness isn't limited to formal meditation sessions; it can be seamlessly integrated into your daily routine. Whether it's savoring a meal together, listening actively during conversations, or taking a moment to appreciate nature during a family walk—everyday activities become opportunities for mindfulness.

MINDFULNESS AND EMOTIONAL REGULATION:

One of the remarkable outcomes of mindfulness is its impact on emotional regulation. As a mindful parent, you're better equipped to navigate your own emotions, modeling healthy emotional expression for your child. This, in turn, fosters their emotional intelligence.

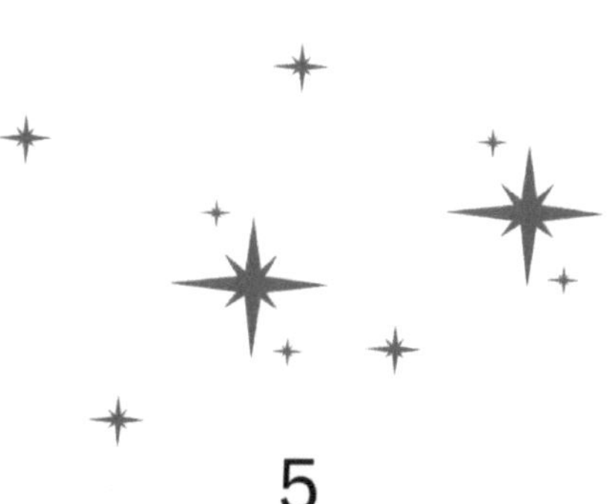

CHAPTER 2: MINDFULNESS DEMYSTIFIED

MINDFULNESS WITH YOUR CHILD:

Extend the benefits of mindfulness to your child by introducing age-appropriate practices. Simple exercises like "mindful breathing" or "mindful listening" can be enjoyable for children and contribute to their overall well-being.

REFLECTION TIME:

Take a moment to reflect on your understanding of mindfulness. How can you incorporate mindfulness into your parenting toolkit? Consider identifying a daily activity where you can intentionally practice being present with your child.

NEXT STEPS:

In the upcoming chapter, we'll explore the science behind mindful parenting, delving into how mindfulness positively influences the brain and emotional well-being. Get ready to uncover the fascinating connections between mindfulness and your parenting journey.

CHAPTER 3: THE SCIENCE BEHIND MINDFUL PARENTING

UNRAVELING THE MINDFUL BRAIN:

As you embrace mindful parenting, it's fascinating to explore the science behind it. Neuroscientific studies reveal that practicing mindfulness can lead to structural changes in the brain, particularly in areas associated with emotional regulation and stress response. Think of it as a workout for the mind, sculpting resilience and calm.

THE AMYGDALA'S DANCE:

Meet the amygdala, the brain's emotional control center. Mindful parenting has a profound impact here, reducing the amygdala's reactivity to stressors. As a result, you become better equipped to respond calmly to challenging parenting moments.

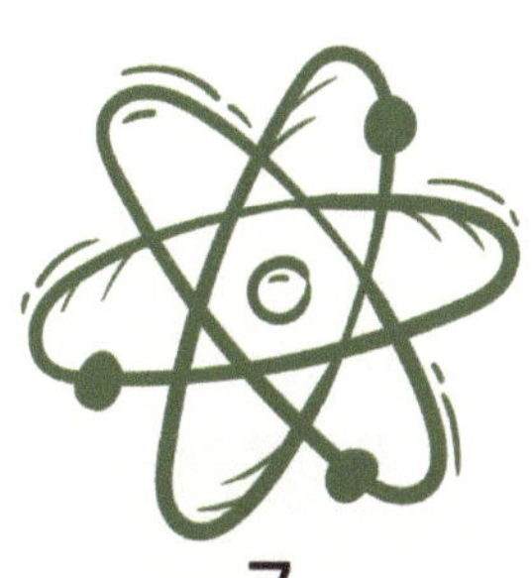

CHAPTER 3: THE SCIENCE BEHIND MINDFUL PARENTING

NEUROPLASTICITY - YOUR BRAIN'S FLEXIBILITY GYM:

Picture your brain as a flexible muscle that adapts to your experiences. Mindfulness, like a workout routine, enhances neuroplasticity—the brain's ability to reorganize itself. This adaptability contributes to improved emotional well-being and resilience.

THE RIPPLE EFFECT ON EMOTIONAL WELL-BEING:

Mindfulness not only impacts your brain but also influences your overall emotional well-being. Studies suggest that regular mindfulness practices contribute to lower levels of stress, anxiety, and depressive symptoms. As a mindful parent, you're fostering a positive emotional environment for both you and your child.

CHAPTER 3: THE SCIENCE BEHIND MINDFUL PARENTING

THE MIRROR NEURONS - CONNECTING PARENT AND CHILD:

Ever heard of mirror neurons? These fascinating neural cells imitate the actions and emotions of others. As a mindful parent, your calm and connected demeanor positively influences your child's emotional regulation through this neural dance.

YOUR MINDFUL TOOLBOX:

Armed with the knowledge of how mindfulness shapes your brain and emotional well-being, envision your mindful toolbox expanding. It's not just a collection of tools; it's a dynamic resource adapting to the evolving landscape of your parenting journey.

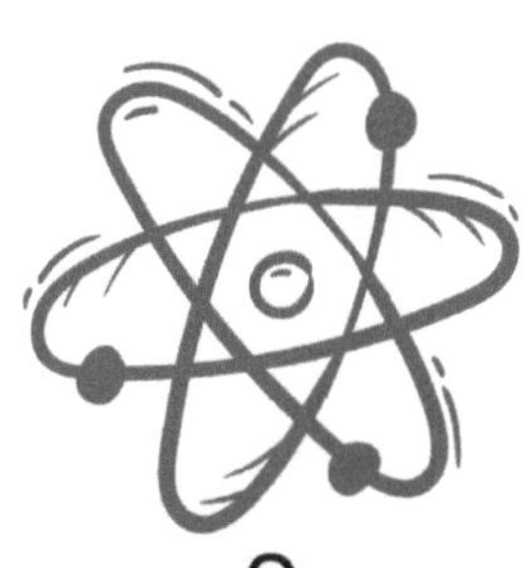

CHAPTER 3: THE SCIENCE BEHIND MINDFUL PARENTING

REFLECTION TIME:

Pause and reflect on the newfound knowledge of the science behind mindfulness. How does understanding the brain's response to mindfulness inspire you to continue your journey of calm and connected parenting?

NEXT STEPS:

In the next chapter, we'll delve into practical strategies for creating mindful moments in your daily life. From mindful breathing to integrating mindfulness into routine activities, get ready to infuse your parenting journey with intentional presence.

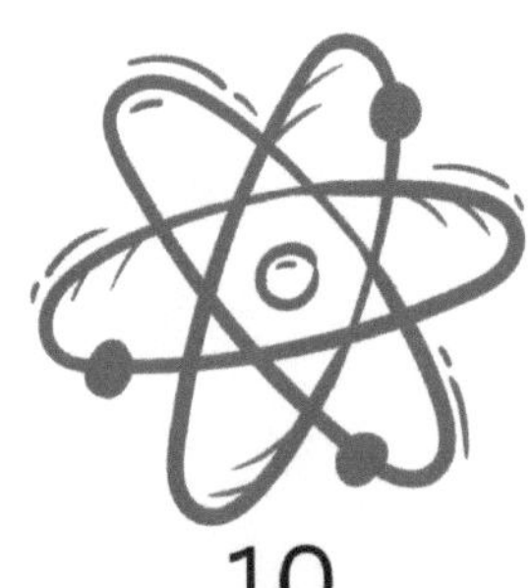

CHAPTER 4: CREATING MINDFUL MOMENTS

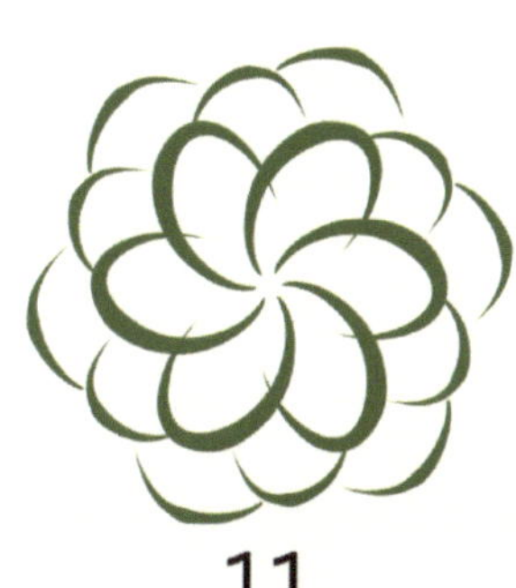

EMBRACING EVERYDAY MINDFULNESS:

Welcome to the art of creating mindful moments in the tapestry of your daily life. Mindfulness is not an abstract concept; it thrives in the ordinary. In this chapter, we'll explore practical strategies to infuse mindfulness into your routines, transforming the mundane into moments of connection and joy.

THE MORNING RITUAL - A MINDFUL START

Imagine your mornings as a canvas waiting to be painted with intention. We'll explore simple yet powerful mindfulness practices to kickstart your day, setting a positive tone for both you and your child. From mindful breathing during breakfast to sharing gratitude, these rituals cultivate a sense of presence.

CHAPTER 4: CREATING MINDFUL MOMENTS

MINDFUL TRANSITIONS - FROM CHAOS TO CALM

Life is a series of transitions, and mindful parenting allows you to navigate them gracefully. Discover how to bring mindfulness into transitional moments like leaving for school, returning home, or transitioning between activities. These intentional pauses become anchors in your day.

MINDFUL MOMENTS IN PLAY:

Playtime isn't just for your child; it's an opportunity for you to be present and engaged. Explore mindful play activities that not only enhance your connection but also bring a sense of joy and laughter to your interactions. From board games to imaginative play, every moment becomes a mindful adventure.

CHAPTER 4: CREATING MINDFUL MOMENTS

MINDFUL MEALTIME CONNECTIONS:

Family meals offer a rich canvas for mindfulness. We'll delve into the art of mindful eating, fostering an appreciation for the sensory experience of food. Learn how to turn mealtime into a moment of connection, conversation, and shared presence.

CREATING YOUR MINDFUL MOMENTS CALENDAR:

As you explore the various ways to infuse mindfulness into your day, consider creating a mindful moments calendar. This visual guide can help you plan intentional pauses, ensuring that moments of connection are woven into the fabric of your daily life.

CHAPTER 4: CREATING MINDFUL MOMENTS

REFLECTION TIME:

Pause and reflect on the mindful moments you've discovered in this chapter. What resonates with you, and how do you envision incorporating these practices into your daily routine?

NEXT STEPS:

In the upcoming chapter, we'll explore mindful breathing techniques—a fundamental practice that anchors you in the present moment. Get ready to unlock the power of your breath in navigating the beautiful chaos of parenthood.

CHAPTER 5: MINDFUL BREATHING TECHNIQUES

THE BREATH AS YOUR ANCHOR:

As we delve into the heart of mindfulness, let's focus on the breath—the ever-present anchor that grounds us in the present moment. In this chapter, we'll explore mindful breathing techniques, simple yet profound practices that serve as your gateway to calm and connected parenting.

MINDFUL BELLY BREATHING:

Start by finding a quiet space, sit comfortably, and place one hand on your chest and the other on your belly. Inhale deeply through your nose, feeling your belly expand like a balloon. Exhale slowly through your mouth, noticing your belly fall. This technique fosters relaxation and brings immediate calm.

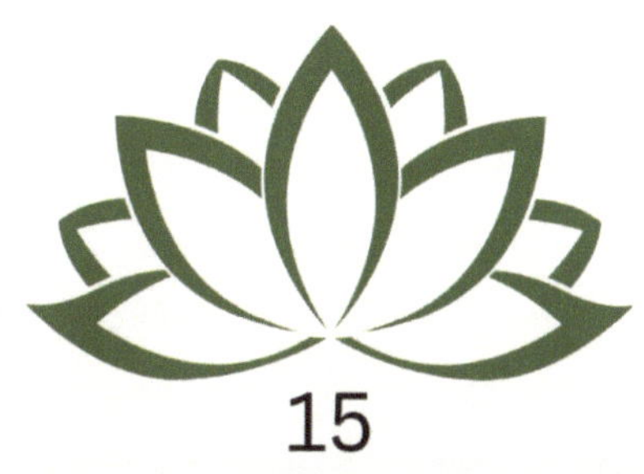

CHAPTER 5: MINDFUL BREATHING TECHNIQUES

4-7-8 TECHNIQUE:

This rhythmic breathing exercise involves inhaling for a count of 4, holding your breath for 7 counts, and exhaling for 8 counts. As you practice, you'll find your body and mind entering a state of deep relaxation. Use this technique during moments of stress or as a prelude to sleep.

BOX BREATHING:

Imagine tracing the sides of a square: inhale for a count of 4, hold your breath for 4 counts, exhale for 4 counts, and then hold your breath again for 4 counts. This structured approach enhances focus, reduces anxiety, and serves as a portable tool for moments of tension.

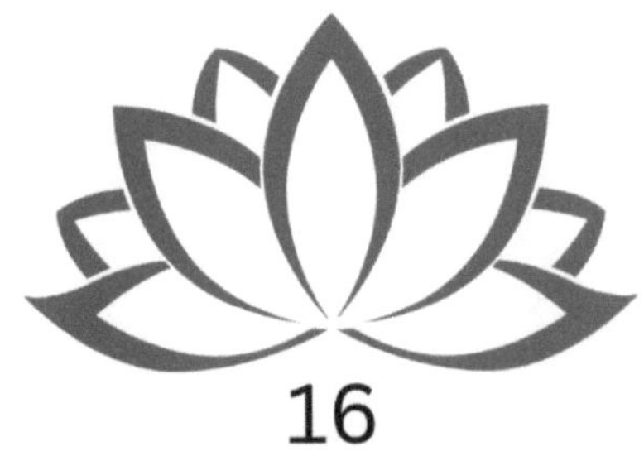

CHAPTER 5: MINDFUL BREATHING TECHNIQUES

MINDFUL BREATHING WITH YOUR CHILD:

Extend the benefits of mindful breathing to your child through interactive activities. Consider creating a "mindful breathing buddy" using a stuffed animal. Guide your child to focus on their breath as they hug their buddy, turning it into a comforting and enjoyable experience.

INTEGRATING MINDFUL BREATHING INTO DAILY LIFE:

Beyond dedicated practice sessions, explore ways to integrate mindful breathing into your daily routine. Whether it's taking a mindful breath before entering your home, during a challenging parenting moment, or before bedtime, these moments of pause become your mindful anchors.

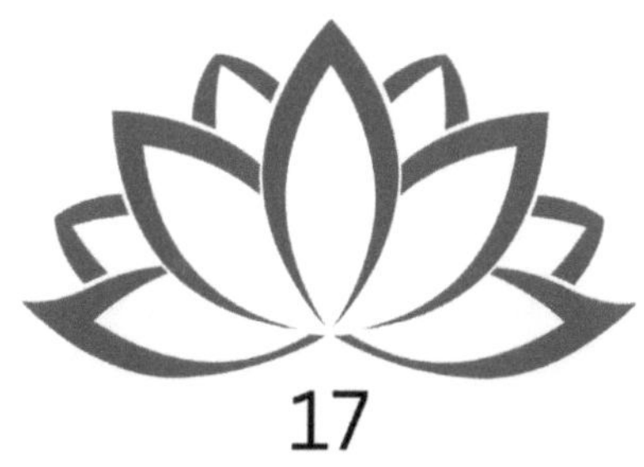

CHAPTER 5: MINDFUL BREATHING TECHNIQUES

REFLECTION TIME:

Take a few mindful breaths and reflect on the experience. How did these breathing techniques impact your sense of calm? Consider incorporating them into your daily routine and observe the ripple effect on your parenting journey.

NEXT STEPS:

In the upcoming chapter, we'll explore the importance of responsive parenting versus reactive parenting. Get ready to cultivate thoughtful responses in the face of parenting challenges.

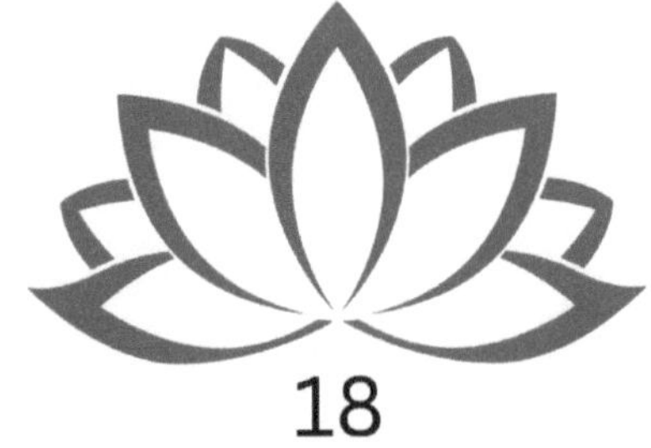

CHAPTER 6: RESPONSIVE PARENTING VS. REACTIVE PARENTING

UNDERSTANDING THE DIFFERENCE:

Welcome to the heart of mindful parenting—distinguishing between reactive and responsive parenting. In this chapter, we'll explore how mindful awareness allows you to step back, evaluate situations, and respond thoughtfully, fostering a deeper connection with your child.

THE REACTIVE RESPONSE:

Picture a typical reactive response: an immediate, instinctive reaction triggered by emotions. While these responses are natural, they may not always align with your parenting goals. Mindful parenting invites you to pause, creating space between the stimulus and your response.

CHAPTER 6: RESPONSIVE PARENTING VS. REACTIVE PARENTING

THE ART OF RESPONSIVENESS:

Responsive parenting involves a thoughtful pause before responding. It's about considering your child's perspective, your emotions, and the context of the situation. This intentional approach allows you to navigate challenges with empathy and understanding.

CREATING THE MINDFUL PAUSE:

Imagine a pause button that gives you the time to collect your thoughts. This is the mindful pause—a momentary break that allows you to choose your response consciously. It can be as simple as taking a breath before addressing a situation.

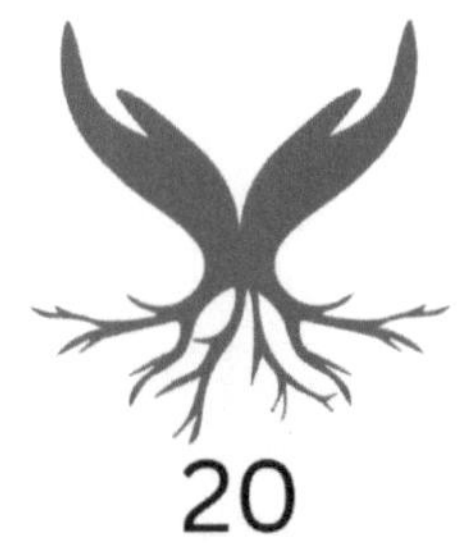

CHAPTER 6: RESPONSIVE PARENTING VS. REACTIVE PARENTING

BUILDING EMPATHY THROUGH MINDFUL RESPONSES:

Mindful responsiveness fosters empathy by acknowledging and validating your child's emotions. As you become attuned to their needs, you strengthen the parent-child connection, creating an environment where they feel heard and understood.

MINDFUL PROBLEM-SOLVING:

Responsive parenting encourages collaborative problem-solving. By involving your child in finding solutions, you empower them to think critically and contribute to the resolution of challenges. This collaborative approach nurtures their confidence and independence.

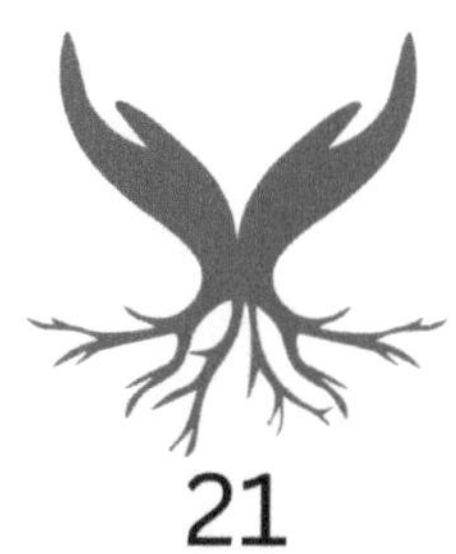

CHAPTER 6: RESPONSIVE PARENTING VS. REACTIVE PARENTING

REFLECTION TIME:

Pause and reflect on a recent parenting situation. How did you respond, and was it reactive or responsive? Consider how implementing mindful pauses and thoughtful responses can transform future interactions.

NEXT STEPS:

In the upcoming chapter, we'll explore practical strategies for managing parental stress mindfully. Get ready to navigate the inevitable challenges of parenting with a calm and centered mindset.

CHAPTER 7: MANAGING PARENTAL STRESS MINDFULLY

THE STRESS PARENTING CONUNDRUM:

Parenthood comes with its fair share of stressors, but the key lies in how you navigate and manage them. In this chapter, we'll delve into mindful strategies to handle parental stress, ensuring that you remain a calm and connected anchor for your child amidst life's inevitable challenges.

RECOGNIZING STRESS TRIGGERS:

The first step in managing parental stress mindfully is identifying the triggers. Whether it's time constraints, unexpected challenges, or the pressure to meet societal expectations, recognizing these stressors allows you to address them proactively.

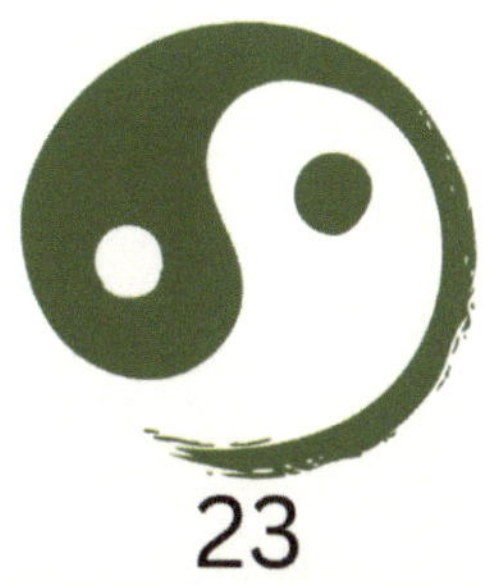

CHAPTER 7: MANAGING PARENTAL STRESS MINDFULLY

THE POWER OF MINDFUL BREATHING IN STRESSFUL MOMENTS:

Revisit the mindful breathing techniques introduced earlier as your go-to tool during stressful moments. A few intentional breaths can create a space for clarity, helping you respond to stress with a composed mindset.

CREATING A MINDFUL STRESS MANAGEMENT PLAN:

Develop a personalized stress management plan that aligns with your lifestyle. This could include daily mindfulness practices, short breaks for self-care, or even seeking support when needed. Your stress management plan is a proactive step toward a more resilient you.

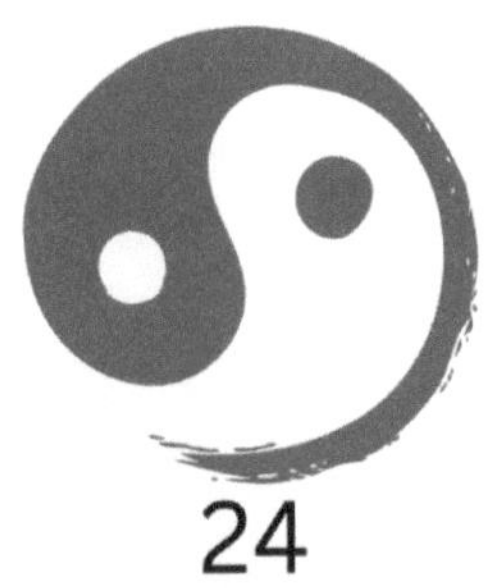

CHAPTER 7: MANAGING PARENTAL STRESS MINDFULLY

THE ART OF LETTING GO:

Mindful parenting involves acknowledging that some stressors are beyond your control. Practice the art of letting go, releasing the burden of perfectionism, and embracing the imperfections that make your parenting journey unique.

MINDFUL MOVEMENT AND EXERCISE:

Physical activity is a powerful stress reducer. Incorporate mindful movement or exercise into your routine. Whether it's a brisk walk, yoga, or dance, movement releases tension and energizes your mind.

CHAPTER 7: MANAGING PARENTAL STRESS MINDFULLY

REFLECTION TIME:

Reflect on your current stress management strategies. What techniques resonate with you, and how might you incorporate mindfulness into your existing plan? Consider creating a mindful stress management toolkit.

NEXT STEPS:

In the upcoming chapter, we'll explore the art of being fully present with your child—cultivating the practice of mindful presence in everyday interactions.

CHAPTER 8: THE ART OF PRESENCE

EMBRACING MINDFUL PRESENCE:

Welcome to the art of being fully present with your child—an essential aspect of mindful parenting. In this chapter, we'll explore the transformative power of mindful presence, fostering deeper connections and savoring the richness of everyday moments.

THE GIFT OF FULL ATTENTION:

Imagine your child sharing a story or achievement, and you, fully engaged, absorbing every detail. This is the gift of full attention. Practice putting aside distractions, be it your phone or other thoughts, and give your child the present of your presence.

MINDFUL LISTENING:

Listening is more than hearing; it's about understanding. Explore the art of mindful listening—tuning in not only to the words but also to the emotions and nuances behind them. This deepens your connection and strengthens the bond with your child.

CHAPTER 8: THE ART OF PRESENCE

BEING PRESENT IN ROUTINE ACTIVITIES:

Transform routine activities into opportunities for connection. Whether it's cooking together, doing homework, or a bedtime routine, approach these moments with mindfulness. Engage in the activity wholeheartedly, turning it into a shared experience.

MINDFUL EYE CONTACT AND NON-VERBAL COMMUNICATION:

Your eyes communicate volumes. Practice mindful eye contact, especially during conversations. It conveys attentiveness, empathy, and love. Non-verbal cues are powerful tools in building a strong emotional connection with your child.

MINDFUL AFFECTION AND TOUCH:

Physical touch is a profound way to express love and connection. Whether it's a hug, a pat on the back, or holding hands, engage in mindful affection. Be present in these moments, savoring the warmth and comfort they bring.

CHAPTER 8: THE ART OF PRESENCE

REFLECTION TIME:

Reflect on recent interactions with your child. Were there moments where you were fully present, and how did it impact the connection between you? Consider one activity where you can practice mindful presence today.

NEXT STEPS:

In the upcoming chapter, we'll explore mindful communication—enhancing the quality of your interactions with your child through thoughtful and empathetic communication.

CHAPTER 9: MINDFUL COMMUNICATION

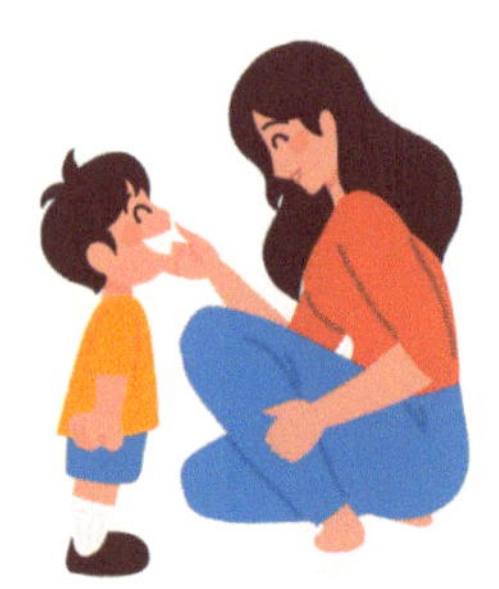

THE HEART OF CONNECTION:

Communication is the bridge that connects hearts and minds. In this chapter, we'll explore the transformative power of mindful communication—building trust, fostering understanding, and creating a nurturing environment for your child to thrive.

THE MINDFUL ART OF SPEAKING:

Consider the words you choose and their impact. Mindful speaking involves expressing yourself with clarity, kindness, and intention. It's about fostering an open and safe space for your child to share their thoughts and feelings.

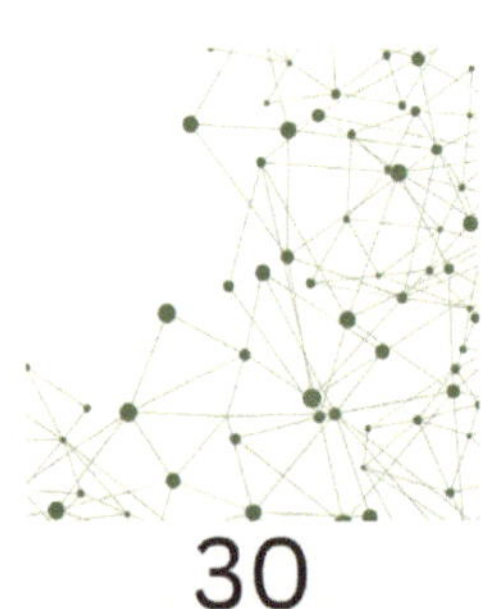

CHAPTER 9: MINDFUL COMMUNICATION

CULTIVATING EMPATHETIC LISTENING:

Empathetic listening goes beyond hearing words; it involves understanding and validating emotions. Practice mindful listening by fully engaging in conversations, withholding judgment, and acknowledging your child's feelings.

ASKING OPEN-ENDED QUESTIONS:

Encourage meaningful conversations by asking open-ended questions. These invite your child to share their thoughts, dreams, and experiences, fostering a deeper connection and understanding of their world.

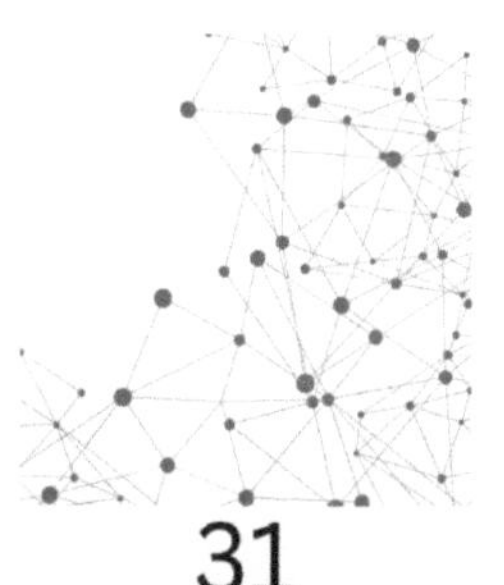

CHAPTER 9: MINDFUL COMMUNICATION

MINDFUL CONFLICT RESOLUTION:

Conflicts are natural in any relationship. Mindful conflict resolution involves approaching disagreements with empathy, active listening, and a collaborative mindset. It's an opportunity for growth and understanding.

THE POWER OF NON-VERBAL COMMUNICATION:

Non-verbal cues, such as body language and facial expressions, play a significant role in communication. Be mindful of your non-verbal signals, as they contribute to the overall tone of your interactions with your child.

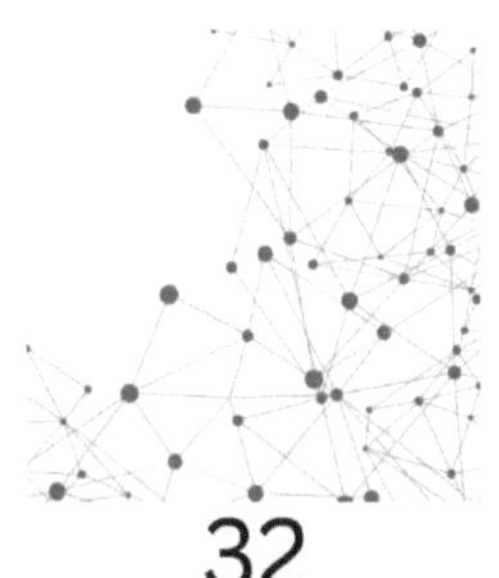

CHAPTER 9: MINDFUL COMMUNICATION

REFLECTION TIME:

Reflect on a recent conversation with your child. How did mindful communication enhance the connection? Consider one aspect of mindful communication you'd like to focus on improving.

NEXT STEPS:

In the upcoming chapter, we'll explore the importance of creating a mindful and harmonious home environment—setting the stage for positive interactions and a sense of calm for the entire family.

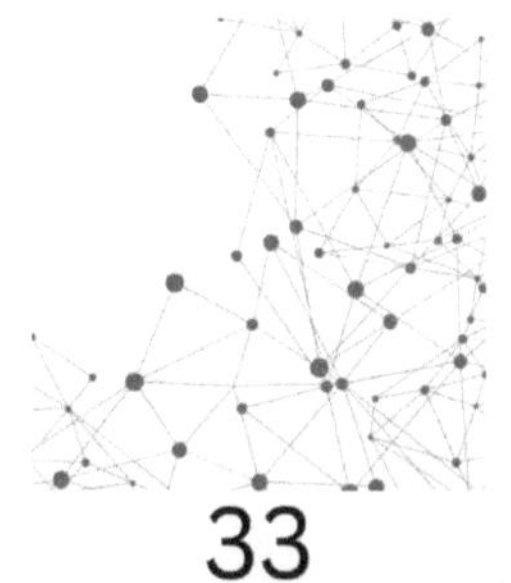

CHAPTER 10: CREATING A MINDFUL HOME ENVIRONMENT

THE SANCTUARY OF HOME:

Your home is more than just a physical space; it's the emotional sanctuary where connections flourish. In this chapter, we'll explore how to infuse mindfulness into your home environment, creating a harmonious and nurturing space for your family.

SIMPLIFYING SPACES FOR SERENITY:

Embrace the principle of simplicity within your home. Decluttering and organizing spaces create an environment that fosters calmness and reduces stress. Invite your child to participate in creating a serene and ordered home.

CHAPTER 10: CREATING A MINDFUL HOME ENVIRONMENT

MINDFUL DESIGN AND COLOR:

Colors and design elements impact mood and energy. Consider incorporating calming colors and elements inspired by nature into your home. Soft blues, greens, and natural textures can contribute to a soothing and mindful atmosphere.

CREATING MINDFUL FAMILY SPACES:

Designate areas within your home for shared activities and quality time. Whether it's a cozy reading nook, a family game table, or a shared cooking space, these areas become focal points for connection and bonding.

CHAPTER 10: CREATING A MINDFUL HOME ENVIRONMENT

MINDFUL TECHNOLOGY USE:

Technology is a part of modern life, but mindful use is key. Establish technology-free zones or times within your home to encourage face-to-face interactions. Create a mindful balance that promotes connection and presence.

ESTABLISHING MINDFUL ROUTINES:

Incorporate mindfulness into daily routines. Whether it's a mindful morning routine, a gratitude practice before bedtime, or a family mindfulness session, these routines cultivate a sense of presence and togetherness.

CHAPTER 10: CREATING A MINDFUL HOME ENVIRONMENT

REFLECTION TIME:

Reflect on the current atmosphere of your home. How can you integrate mindful elements into your living space to create a more serene and connected environment? Consider one change you can make this week.

NEXT STEPS:

In the upcoming chapter, we'll explore the significance of mindful rituals and traditions—ceremonies that weave a tapestry of connection, memories, and joy within your family.

CHAPTER 11: MINDFUL RITUALS AND TRADITIONS

THE HEARTBEAT OF FAMILY LIFE:

Rituals and traditions are the heartbeat of family life, weaving a tapestry of shared experiences, connection, and joy. In this chapter, we'll explore the significance of mindful rituals and traditions, creating lasting memories that anchor your family.

THE POWER OF CONSISTENCY:

Mindful rituals provide a sense of stability and consistency in the ever-changing landscape of family life. Whether it's a weekly family game night or a monthly nature outing, these regular rituals become anticipated and cherished moments.

CHAPTER 11: MINDFUL RITUALS AND TRADITIONS

INFUSING MEANING INTO TRADITIONS:

Mindful traditions carry meaning and significance. Reflect on the values and messages you want to impart through your family traditions. Whether it's celebrating cultural heritage, expressing gratitude, or fostering kindness, infuse intention into your traditions.

CELEBRATING MILESTONES MINDFULLY:

Marking milestones is a celebration of growth and shared accomplishments. Mindful celebrations focus on the essence of the milestone, fostering a sense of achievement, connection, and the anticipation of future adventures.

CHAPTER 11: MINDFUL RITUALS AND TRADITIONS

NATURE AS A MINDFUL BACKDROP:

Consider incorporating nature into your family rituals and traditions. Whether it's a mindful nature walk, a camping trip, or a garden planting ceremony, nature provides a serene backdrop for creating lasting memories.

MINDFUL HOLIDAY CELEBRATIONS:

Holidays are opportunities to create lasting memories. Approach holiday celebrations with mindfulness—focusing on connection, gratitude, and shared joy. These mindful celebrations become cherished memories for your child.

CHAPTER 11: MINDFUL RITUALS AND TRADITIONS

REFLECTION TIME:

Reflect on the current rituals and traditions within your family. How can you infuse more mindfulness into these moments to deepen connection and create lasting memories? Consider one mindful addition to a current tradition or the introduction of a new one.

NEXT STEPS:

In the upcoming chapter, we'll explore strategies for overcoming challenges and maintaining a mindful parenting mindset. Get ready to navigate the inevitable obstacles with resilience and presence.

CHAPTER 12: OVERCOMING CHALLENGES MINDFULLY

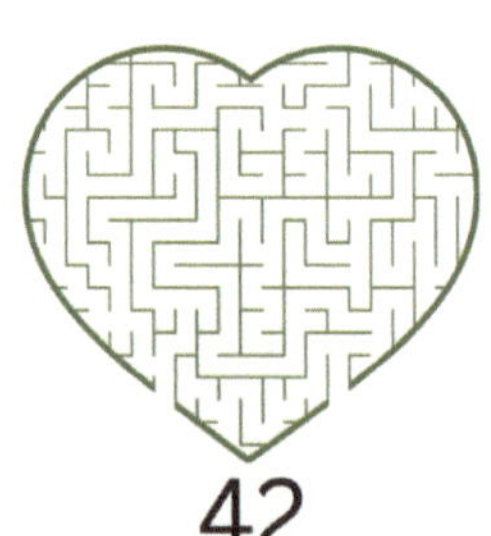

THE DANCE OF CHALLENGES:

In the dance of parenthood, challenges are inevitable. In this chapter, we'll explore mindful strategies for navigating obstacles, cultivating resilience, and maintaining a positive parenting mindset in the face of adversity.

EMBRACING IMPERFECTION:

Mindful parenting acknowledges that imperfection is a part of the journey. Embrace the messiness of life, learn from challenges, and recognize that each stumble is an opportunity for growth—for both you and your child.

CHAPTER 12: OVERCOMING CHALLENGES MINDFULLY

MINDFUL PROBLEM-SOLVING:

Approach challenges with a mindful problem-solving mindset. Break down the issue into manageable parts, involve your child in finding solutions, and celebrate the small victories along the way. This collaborative approach fosters resilience.

THE POWER OF SELF-COMPASSION:

Extend the same compassion to yourself that you offer to your child. Parenting is a learning journey, and mistakes are inevitable. Practice self-compassion, allowing room for growth and self-improvement without self-judgment.

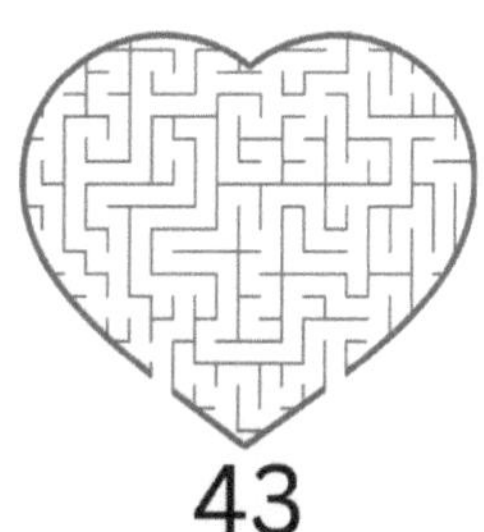

CHAPTER 12: OVERCOMING CHALLENGES MINDFULLY

MINDFUL TIME MANAGEMENT:

Balancing the demands of parenthood requires mindful time management. Prioritize tasks, set realistic expectations, and allow flexibility. Mindful time management ensures that you allocate time for both responsibilities and meaningful moments with your child.

SEEKING SUPPORT MINDFULLY:

Recognize when you need support and seek it mindfully. Whether it's from friends, family, or parenting communities, sharing challenges and learning from others enhances your resilience and provides valuable perspectives.

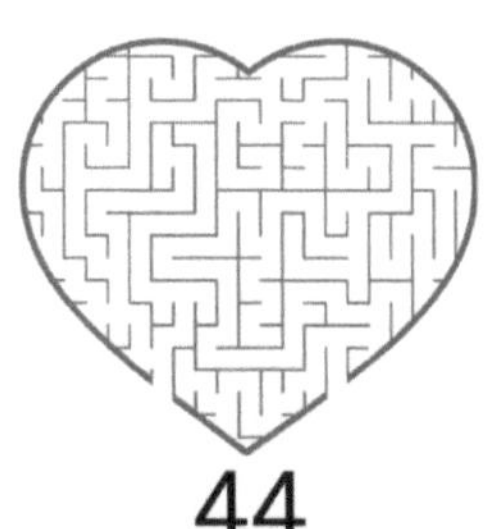

CHAPTER 12: OVERCOMING CHALLENGES MINDFULLY

REFLECTION TIME:

Reflect on a recent parenting challenge. How did you navigate it, and what mindful strategies did you employ? Consider one area where you can implement a mindful approach to overcome challenges more effectively.

NEXT STEPS:

In the final chapter, we'll reflect on the mindful parenting journey and explore ways to continue nurturing a strong, connected, and joyful relationship with your child.

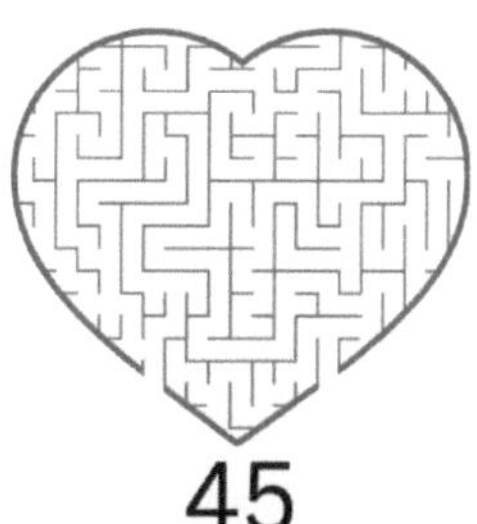

CHAPTER 13: EMBRACING THE MINDFUL PARENTING JOURNEY

REFLECTING ON THE JOURNEY:

As we approach the culmination of this mindful parenting guide, take a moment to reflect on the journey you've embarked upon. Celebrate the progress, acknowledge the challenges, and recognize the transformative power of mindfulness in your parenting experience.

NURTURING CONNECTION AND JOY:

Mindful parenting is a continuous journey of nurturing connection and joy. Consider the moments of laughter, shared experiences, and the deepening bond with your child. These are the treasures that make the journey worthwhile.

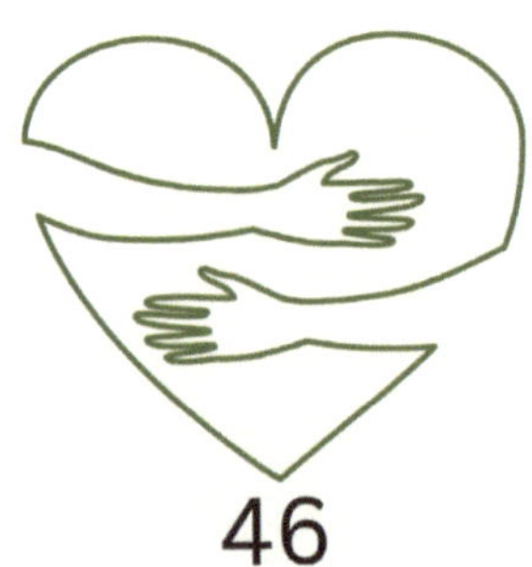

CHAPTER 13: EMBRACING THE MINDFUL PARENTING JOURNEY

SETTING INTENTIONS FOR THE FUTURE:

As you look ahead, set mindful intentions for your parenting journey. What aspects of mindful parenting do you want to continue cultivating? How can you further enhance the connection with your child and create lasting memories?

THE EVER-EVOLVING DANCE:

Parenting, like life, is an ever-evolving dance. Embrace the beauty of growth and change—both in yourself and your child. Mindfulness provides the compass for navigating this dynamic dance with grace and presence.

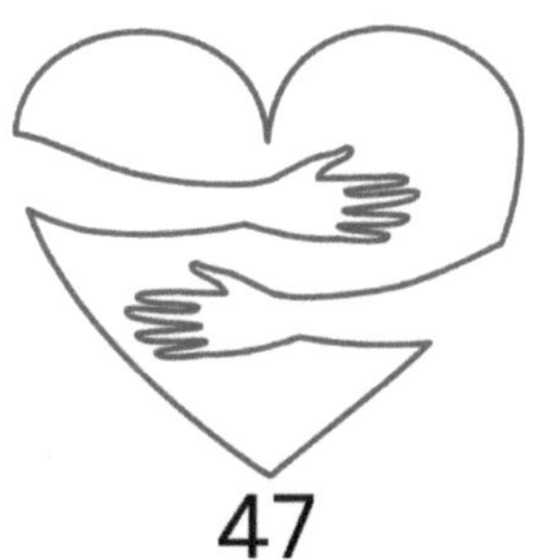

CHAPTER 13: EMBRACING THE MINDFUL PARENTING JOURNEY

GRATITUDE FOR THE PRESENT:

Express gratitude for the present moment. Amidst the busyness of life, savor the small victories, the shared smiles, and the everyday magic that unfolds within your family. Gratitude anchors you in the richness of the now.

CONTINUING THE MINDFUL PARENTING LEGACY:

Consider the legacy you're creating through mindful parenting. The lessons of presence, empathy, and resilience will ripple through generations. Your commitment to mindful parenting becomes a cherished gift to your child and future generations.

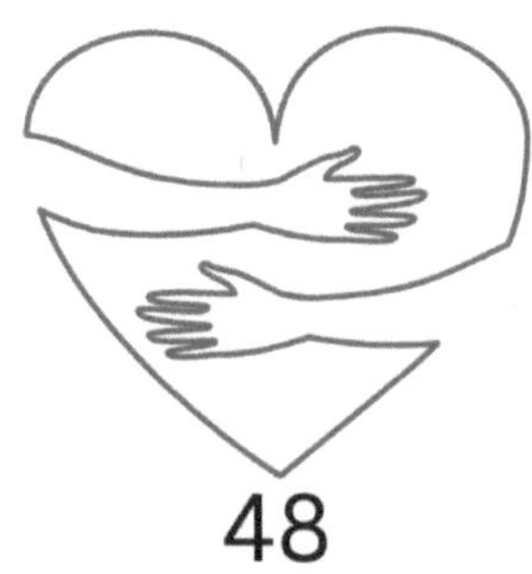

CHAPTER 13: EMBRACING THE MINDFUL PARENTING JOURNEY

CONCLUSION:

As we conclude this guide, remember that mindful parenting is not a destination but a lifelong journey. Your commitment to being present, fostering connection, and navigating challenges mindfully lays the foundation for a strong and joyful parent-child relationship.

Thank you for allowing ThoughtHarbor Publishing to be a part of your mindful parenting journey. May your days be filled with love, connection, and the beauty of mindful presence.

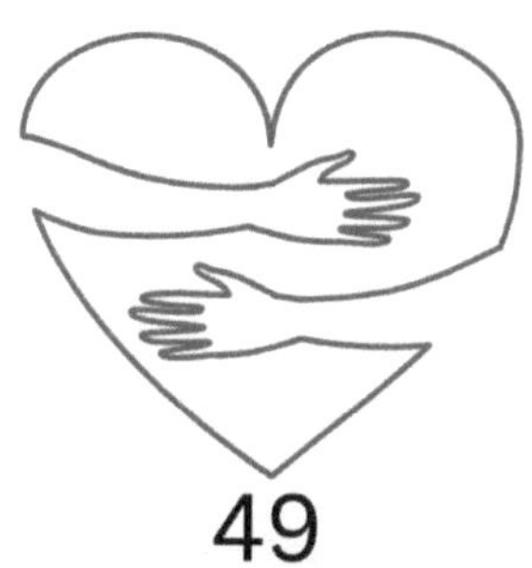

THANK YOU!

As we wrap up "Calm and Connected: Navigating Parenthood Mindfully," a big thank you for being part of this mindful parenting adventure with ThoughtHarbor Publishing. Together, we've explored how to be more present, communicate better, and create a mindful home for your family.

Remember, mindful parenting is a lifelong journey filled with small victories and shared moments.

As you keep growing together with your child, embrace imperfections, celebrate progress, and cherish each moment. May the wisdom shared here be a helpful guide on your parenting path, creating a home filled with love, understanding, and support.

Thanks for choosing ThoughtHarbor Publishing as your mindful parenting companion. Here's to more peaceful and connected moments in your family!

Warm wishes,
Cristian Secrieru

ThoughtHarbor Publishing